The Panacea Cleanse

"A Powerful, 12-Day, Plant Based Detoxification and Healing Guide: Complete with Recipes and Shopping Lists"

Nathan Crane

The Panacea Cleanse

By; Nathan Crane

This book is dedicated to all of the teachers in my life

who have given me guidance, light, energy, and love.

CONTENTS

Welcome to the Panacea Cleanse

I congratulate you for taking this exciting step of committing yourself to this complete mind, body, and spirit cleanse. I will tell you straight-out that it is both a challenging, yet extremely rewarding and life-changing experience.

Whether you've done any type of cleanse in the past, or this is your first one, I commend you for taking this action in wanting to become healthier, happier, and more energetic in your life.

After having experimented with my very first master-cleanse years ago, I became intrigued and interested in figuring out which types of cleanses are the least harmful and most healthful to the human body.

I wanted to know if there was a cleanse available that would be safe, healthy, raw, natural, and organic that didn't take your body through instant levels of extreme changes, as most cleanses out there do.

I've tried cleansing with capsules and formulas sold at health food stores. I've tried master-cleanses, water cleanses, juice cleanses, and psyllium husk cleanses. After experimenting with dozens of cleanses from all different types of cultures, I came to the realization that although the various cleanses were beneficial to my body, none of the cleanses I had taken were designed with the purest essence of nature in mind.

While all of the cleanses I tried did have their benefits and advantages, none of them helped my body, mind, and spirit achieve it's natural, purified, healthy state of self-healing.

The capsules and formulas you can buy online and at the store are convenient, but they don't cleanse your brain and mind of their perpetual toxins, and they don't help you break bad eating habits that caused you to need to cleanse yourself in the first place.

Many cleanses that I've tried are too extreme on your body and take you from an extremely unhealthy state, to a seemingly healthy one, but unfortunately it doesn't give your body all the nutrients and support it needs to truly cleanse out all the toxins stored within your cells, while rejuvenating your mind and spirit at the same time.

So after studying, testing, and experimenting with all these different types of cleanses, I finally came to the realization that I needed to figure out a cleanse that would rejuvenate my body, cleanse the toxins, break bad eating habits, lose weight, and purify my mind, body, and spirit on a deeper level.

I began combining the different elements of each cleanse until I figured out a cleansing plan that would help me achieve a higher level of health, fight dis-eases, and feel great during and after the cleanse as well. I put them all together and then tested, tweaked, and enhanced every element of the cleanse. After experiencing incredible results with my wife and myself, I decided there was no better name to give it than; The Panacea Cleanse.

Panacea, pronounced Pan-a-sea, is a Greek word which means "The cure to all dis-eases." This cleanse was designed to help put your body into a state of self-healing where you can begin to ward of any ailments you may be experiencing. Once the body is put into this natural state of self-healing, it has the capability to make miracles happen.

When your body is being cleansed of all the toxins and being fed by the right nutrients, it has the potential to overcome any and all dis-eases you may be feeling. While the cleanse is extremely important, the follow-up lifestyle and habit changing diet, which we will get into later in this book, is just as important as well.

Being an avid student of hypnosis, auto-induction, and auto-suggestion, I've come to realize that by putting your brain into a state that allows it to send healing signals to your body, it will help you become more conscious, healthy, and self-healed, automatically. As a bonus to this cleanse, I've created an audio that you can listen to each night before sleeping that will help you cleanse your mind, body, and spirit naturally, quickly, and effectively.

You can download this audio along with additional videos that walk you through every step of the cleanse at either www.ThePanaceaCleanse.com, or receive access to them along with other materials when you become a Student of Life at www.ThePanaceaCommunity.com.

FAQs

What if I'm pregnant? My wife did this cleanse while breastfeeding and did extremely well. When a baby is in the mother's body he/she feeds on whatever the mother takes into her body. This cleanse is packed with nutrients as well as cleanses out toxins from the blood stream which is beneficial to the mother and the baby. It is recommended to take Option 2 of the Liver/Gallbladder Cleanse at the end of Day 3 if you are pregnant or if you are experiencing any negative reactions to Epsom Salt.

Make sure you check with your doctor before doing this cleanse.

What if I'm taking medication? Most medication has negative side effects on your body - over time your body gets acquainted with those side affects as well as building immunity to the medication. If you immediately stop taking all medication it's possible to have negative reactions as your body might need to be weaned off of them. Many physicians don't believe in natural cleanses so they may tell you to avoid them, but many people have had positive results from cleansing and have even come off their medication completely after certain periods of cleansing and dietary change. Listening to your body and your intuition will tell you if you're ready to come off the medication. If you plan to wean off your medication or have any doubts about it, you can consult with your physician.

What dis-eases can this cleanse help with? In my personal experience this cleanse has helped me get rid of excess fat cells, cleanse away pimples, expel gallstones, and have a healthier piece of mind about life and diet. While I can not make any claims about this cleanse, I would love to hear how it helps you. Remember, when you cleanse toxins out of your body and rebuild your cells with life-giving nutrients found in nature, miracles can happen and your body can fight and overcome any ailment you may be experiencing.

Can I workout during the cleanse. I typically work out during every cleanse. Working out can help your body cleanse out toxins faster through your sweat glands.

Will I be hungry during the cleanse? Hunger pangs

can occur as a natural process of eliminating whole meals from your diet for a period of time. During my experience in cleansing I have noticed that the hunger pangs often disappear within 72 hours of starting the cleanse.

Do I get protein and other vital nutrients from this cleanse? Yes. The recipes in this cleanse are full of a tremendous amount of vitamins, minerals, amino acids, proteins, antioxidants, and vital nutrients to help your body achieve a higher state of self-healing.

What can I eat during the cleanse?   The recipes are all laid out inside the cleanse. Try to follow them as closely as you can. You will be receiving all of your nutrients in liquid form. Liquid is the fastest way to absorb the nutrients from the food into your bloodstream.

Is this cleanse safe? The Panacea Cleanse was created with safety as it's #1 priority. After experimenting with dozens of cleanses from multiple backgrounds, The Panacea Cleanse helps your body ease in and out of the cleansing process safely and effectively. If you ever have any doubts about doing a cleanse, you can always consult with your physician or health practitioner.

What if I'm vegan? The cleansing recipes in The Panacea Cleanse are raw, organic, and vegan.

Is the cleanse gluten free? Yes.

What will I need to complete the cleanse? This cleanse requires a juicer and a blender. Any type will work.

What if I have questions? You may contact us at any time by sending an email to info@thepanaceacommunity.com with the subject line titled; "The Panacea Cleanse."

Chapter 1. The Panacea Cleanse

The Panacea Cleanse is a full mind, body, and spirit cleanse that is derived from the best elements of nature to help your body reach a state of self-healing and self-understanding so you can change harmful everyday human-habits that cause dis-ease, death, pain, and suffering, to good habits that invoke harmony, health, happiness, and wealth.

I've designed this cleanse to be raw, organic, natural, vegan, and gluten free.

It is a cleanse designed for the majority of the population. As long as you stick your mind to it, follow it step by step, and don't give up, you will begin experiencing the amazing results that myself and others have had the great pleasure of experiencing.

This cleanse may change the way you treat your body forever, and I'll explain why in a minute, but first this is probably a good point to mention that, "I AM NOT A

DOCTOR."

I have no "traditional schooling" in medicine, I am not certified, I AM NOT A PHD. I do not guarantee that this will cure any disease, and I, nor my companies and affiliates, do not take any risk for your actions. This is strictly informational advice and I truly believe in it and I truly believe it can and will help you totally cleanse your mind, body, and spirit, but unfortunately I can not guarantee anything and I expect you to take caution and use common sense when you do this cleanse, or any cleanse for that matter.

I carefully lay out in this book in the FAQ section and in my videos precautionary steps to take if you are on medication or if you are having serious dis-eases and illnesses. I do recommend that if you have any doubts that you may consult with your physician or nutritionist before doing this cleanse, but at the same time I recommend you simply learn how to follow what your body tells you that it needs and listen to the internal advice that comes from within your heart.

Here's the hardcore reality; one out of four people in the

United States has cancer, and that rate is growing every day. Millions of children are becoming overweight and obese before they even reach an age where they make reasonable decisions on their own. Millions of people have diabetes, Alzheimer's, arthritis, and many other diseases every single year.

The unfortunate truth about all of these dis-eases and painful experiences that most humans are experiencing today is that they are completely man-made. The creator did not put dis-eases on the earth so that humans could get pain from them, humans created those dis-eases by manipulating the simple elements of nature into dis-ease causing mutated cellular compounds.

If we want to believe that the devil created these dis-eases, then we would be blind to the fact that when we use the name devil, we are actually referring to our own human-race.

There are definitely dark forces at play that help human-beings make dreadful decisions that cause pain, suffering, and death to our societies, but in the end, it all comes down to our own capacity to choose our own thoughts and make our own decisions.

If we wish to make a positive change in our communities and around our world, we must first start by taking back the control of our minds and not letting other's around us make our decisions for us. We must begin by cleansing our minds and our bodies of the toxins we've filled them up with for centuries so they can become purified and so that we will be able to receive the consciousness that the creator has established for us.

Through the cleansing process, you clean out your rusted pipes which have been attracting dirt and grime for years so that you may be receptive to the thought patterns that are in alignment with the creator. The creator wants us to be healthy, happy, and joyful, but it is us who must make the decisions to do so.

It is many of our scientists who have been changing the structural makeup of our plants, our trees, our food, and our water in an effort to make it last longer, sell for a cheaper price, and be stored and shipped by the tons. They add protons, take away neutrons, mix compounds, mutate cells, and transmutate the natural healing structure that was created for perfect health, into a cellular disaster that eats away the antibodies and cells inside our bodies.

We must put a stop to this and begin by deciding to not only eat organic, kosher, healthy, natural food, but we must not allow human beings to add body-destroying chemicals, fertilizers, pesticides, and toxins to our food. We must not allow our fellow humans to genetically modify food for their own special interests of profits and financial growth.

The future of our planet remains in our hands, our decisions, and our actions, and we must take the steps necessary to achieve a state of human health and cleanliness so that we may drink the life-giving water that runs from our rivers and eat the health-creating naturally organic plants that grow in our forests, once again.

Have you ever sat down to consider exactly what it is that causes human-beings to experience dis-ease? Did you ever take the time to contemplate the cause of cancer, diabetes, arthritis, or any other destructive dis-eases?

Dis-ease means that something is out of balance. It means that something with your mind, body, or spirit is out of alignment with its true natural healing condition. This can be proven to yourself by yourself when you utilize your logic in determining the reasons behind dis-ease. Scientists can prove that every thought, every human, every mind is interconnected. They might not be able to understand it or explain it, but they can prove it, and that's important for humans to understand.

The interconnectedness that runs through our minds, bodies, and spirits can be measured in frequencies and vibrations. Most people call it energy. One of my teachers calls it "thought particles." The aura around the body that people are so amazed with, in his words, could be called "the mind field." The thoughts that we "think" get attracted into the mind field by a naturally occurring magnetic force.

Every thought has an effect somewhere on the planet, and while one thought may not seem like it had any impact, I assure you that every thought, no matter the size, affects not only the entire planet and everything and everybody living on it, but it affects the entire Universe as well.

This interconnectedness that our scientists call energy is really "thought particles" vibrating at different speeds connecting everybody and everything together as one. When we look at why people experience dis-ease, there is only 5 reasons. If we as a human race were able to avoid these 5 things that cause human dis-ease, I am confident that we would not experience any dis-ease at all ever in our lives.

The 5 reasons why a human would experience any dis-ease in the mind, body, or spirit is if:

1. You experience bad or harmful thoughts.
2. You experience bad or harmful emotions.
3. You eat bad or harmful foods.
4. You drink bad or harmful liquids.
5. You take bad or harmful substances (drugs, medication, alcohol, cigarettes, chemicals).

Thoughts and emotions are the number one and number two cause of dis-ease. Here is simple proof for you to grasp. Depression is prevalent around the world today.

Many people are feeling alone, afraid, and sad. They eat until they are over-full and then they gain weight. These people eat quickly and abundantly, hoping they will begin to feel better by avoiding their negative emotions.

While they do feel better for a short period of time, the food-high wears off and the feelings of depression worsen due to the chemicals in the food they have eaten. Therefore these people continue to stay overweight and obese eventually getting the dis-ease of diabetes, or the dis-ease of cancer, or heart dis-ease, or any other dis-eases destroying our humanity today.

Many Doctors will tell you to get your stomach stapled or to take medication to help lose the weight or mask the depression, but what they don't realize is that they are not helping you uncover the number one cause of your eating habits in the first place, and that is your thoughts.

Additionally if you are one of those people like myself who had parents and grandparents who did all of these five dis-ease creating actions in their lives, then you could have been automatically pre-disposed to having dis-eases in your body. But not to worry, all of that can be corrected. With the right nutrition, cleansing, mental activities, and emotional balances, I truly believe that you can cure any and all illnesses known to man and woman.

Your mind, body, and spirit is designed by the Creator to have every single self-healing cell within it's structure so that no matter what dis-ease it experiences, it can correct itself, modify the cellular structure, eliminate the waste, and become healthy and harmonious once again.

I also want to mention that whenever I say "cure," it is because I truly believe that your body and mind can cure itself if given the right opportunity to do so. The reason medical doctors have not been able to cure their patients with drugs and radiation is because they do not put the body into a state of "natural curability." They use science instead of nature. Science only prolongs the day when humans realize that the power of healing is already perfect in it's natural form.

Scientists have told us that bananas have Potassium and oranges have Vitamin C, which both are good for protecting against free-radicals and rejuvenating the cells. But do we really need scientists to tell us what already exists? Are we not smart enough to pay attention to what we put into our bodies and understand the affects it has on us?

Adding drugs, radiation, and chemicals to a disease-stricken body, even if it helps one symptom, will create an onslaught of other symptoms in its place. That's why I do not recommend drugs for any person. There is a time and place for assistance by medical Doctors, such as when you had a terrible accident and lost your leg and they need to stop the bleeding and replace your blood, but those are far and few between, besides, how many people go to the Doctor for an earache, or a headache, or a stomach ache, or a cold? Far too many. And what do the Doctors tell them? "Take this medication which has X, X, and X side effects, and you'll feel better in a few days. If you don't feel better, come back and we'll try something else."

If people only knew that they can heal themselves of any and all ailments simply by the correct use of the natural elements given to us by the creator… oh what a different society we could live in.

In my opinion, most doctors truly think they are helping their patients when they recommend their subscriptions, but the schooling system in place that teaches doctors that medicinal drugs is the way to treat their patients, is not truthful.

The last time I went to the hospital was because I suffered a very uncomfortable injury. I was playing basketball and jumped up as high as I could to block the shot of the offender. He did a pump fake and as soon as I was up in the air, he rammed his shoulder into my hip flipping me upside down.

My body went out of control and began plummeting towards the solid wood floor. In the blink of an eye I was able to turn my body enough so that I wouldn't land on my head, and instead, all of my weight crushed into my right shoulder, slamming the rest of my body on the ground quickly after.

I looked over to my right shoulder in shock and saw that it was out of place. The bone was shooting towards the sky like a boulder emerging from the ground.

At first I thought my shoulder was dislocated. So in my stubborn desire to fix it and keep going on with life, I insisted on somebody in the gym to "pop it" back into place.

Fortunately there was no one there stupid enough at the time to do such an outrageous act, and my wife walked in just in time to swoop me up and drive me to the hospital.

The pain didn't kick in until the shock wore off, and as soon as we arrived at the hospital, the adrenaline dissipated and my entire right arm was plagued by excruciating pain.

After the doctor examined my shoulder and took x-rays, he told me I separated the AC joint. It was a good thing that no one tried popping it back in place because that would have made it much, much worse.

But in the end, what was the doctor's solution? A couple of painkillers and a shoulder sling that ended up costing me $2,250.00. I couldn't even take the painkillers because I had been cleansing my body for a couple of years at that point, and the first painkiller I took made me sick to my stomach. So I dealt with the pain mentally, which to be honest was easier than dealing with the sickness that came from the painkillers.

Nearly a year later my shoulder was still sticking up out of my skin. Why? That injury is considered a dis-ease because it put my mind and body at a dis-comfort, or at dis-ease.

If I would have waited to see a naturopath or someone who has experience in chiropractic, I may have saved myself a lot of money and probably a lot of arthritic problems later. But those are the hard lessons we often get the chance to learn from in life.

So the point is that although we may have been educated by a system that profits from our dis-eases, there are other options available, such as this cleanse, which are designed to help your mind, body, and spirit get into a state of purity so it can begin the healing and curing process all by itself.

I quit drinking hard liquor and beer after many years of abuse with the thanks to this epiphany, and I share it with you in hopes that you may feel the intensity I felt the day it entered my mind;

"to purify the mind, we must purify the body, and to purify the body, we must also purify the mind."

So throughout your cleanses in life, whether this one or another, you will find many opportunities to cheat, go back to old ways, and get back into bad habits. But I implore you not to do so.

I ask that you continue with the cleanse and the daily healthy living plan diligently and with faith and determination.

YOU will be the one who gets to experience the benefits of living a healthy, energetic, happy life. The reward will be greater than a trophy, a prize, or even money. The reward will be a long, healthy, happy life that you get to enjoy with yourself and your family.

Chapter 2. What to Expect

During this cleanse you may experience certain feelings that maybe you never experienced before. You may feel extremely blissful and joyful at times, and you may feel annoyed and even some pain or nausea at others. There is a chance that you feel out-of-body experiences. You might feel like you've left the earth. You might experience epiphanies, laugh attacks, bursts of joy, or spouts of rage.

Your feelings all depend on the level of cleansing that your mind, body, and spirit are experiencing, and it all depends on the amount of mental and physical toxins that are being expelled.

Think of it this way. If you spent twenty years of your life putting toxins into your mind and body, how long do you think it would take to get rid of those toxins?

The logical answer is "a long time", right? Well fortunately that's not the case for everyone. For some people it's going to be much sooner than others, which could only be a matter of days, weeks, or months, and fo others it may take a bit longer. It all really depends on how much effort and discipline you are willing to put into this cleanse and the practice that follows thereafter.

To be honest, it's quite possible that after doing this cleanse once, you will begin to feel and notice amazing results in your mind and your body, and possibly even ge rid of any and all dis-eases and ailments that you were experiencing beforehand.

I know we mentioned out-of-body experiences a moment ago. If you're wondering what an out-of-body experience is, it is basically a moment in time where you enter into a different dimension within the mind and slightly, or entirely disconnect from your physical level of consciousness, taking you into a level of self-hypnosis and deep spiritual connection.

This level of self-hypnosis, or "mind-connection" as one of my teachers Mr Gaitan calls it, can be used as a very powerful tool. During this experience you may feel like five minutes passed when actually it has been hours; or vice versa. You lose consciousness of time.

You may come back to consciousness with new levels of awareness, knowledge and understanding. Or you might just feel relaxed and rejuvenated. It all really just depends on what frequency in the mind you connect to during this experience.

The purpose of this cleanse and the audio and videos that are available with it is to help direct you into the right frequencies in your mind so when you connect to your internal source, you will get the most benefit possible.

Meditation is a great tool; the only problem that occurs for most people when trying meditation is that they have no idea where to connect or how to connect to the frequencies that can help them receive the most benefit.

Meditation, when used properly, can help you control the mind so you can establish a deeper connection while directing your mind to achieve greater mental and physical results.

The audio track will help you do this. So listening to it

diligently will help you develop the right mind connection so you can get the maximum benefit from this cleanse. I by chance you're not able to get access to the audios, don't worry, you will still be able to receive incredible benefits from completing the cleanse laid out herein all by itself.

I'd also like to point out that if you feel any headaches, it is usually because you are dehydrated, and you simply need to drink more water.

Water is actually the greatest cleanser this earth has to offer, and the more water, preferably fresh spring water, we drink, the greater ability our bodies will have to facilitate the cleansing process.

Chapter 3. The Power of Water

You will notice that during the days you are cleansing, the most important thing your body needs is water.

You can live for weeks and even months without food, but without water you could die in a week. The cells of your body are filled with water, covering nearly 70% of our cellular structure and nearly the same percentage of the earth. There is a very specific purpose for this phenomena and it's something to pay close attention to and contemplate upon.

The major problem with water today is that we are basically destroying it with all the poisons we dump down the drains. You might not think about it, but when we use commercial shampoos and soaps, even when they portray the misleading term "natural," they are made from many different harmful chemicals that enter the water, and later come right back into the water that we put back into our bodies.

Many companies will trick you when they tell you "Vitamin E" healthy shampoo or "Vitamin B Natural soap". Many times if you read the labels on the back of these soaps and shampoos you will see that they are filled with processed chemicals that not only enter your skin, the largest organ on your body, every single time you use them, but later go into the drains and come back into your washing or drinking water as well.

If you continue to use shampoos and soaps that are filled with hidden chemicals, those chemicals will seep into the pores of your skin and enter your bloodstream, eventually causing you physical problems later on in life.

You might ask how these companies are able to sell this soap that causes harm to the human body, but the reality is that most of our food, cosmetics, soaps, conditioners, cleaning supplies, toothpastes, medicine, and prescriptions are all composed of harmful chemicals that hurt the human body.

The only way to put an end to this madness is to start taking action one person at a time and start using pure, organic, soaps, shampoos, cleaners, foods, juices, and toothpastes.

We as human beings are the only ones who create the demand for these products, and as long as we increase our level of consciousness and take action to get the products that are most beneficial to our minds and bodies, the companies will eventually have to fill that demand.

The shampoo I love and have used for years now, that my curly haired wife also uses and loves, is the best multi-purpose shampoo, cleaning soap, body scrub, laundry detergent, and face cleansing soap I have ever used.

It comes in many different variations of smells and flavors, and it is made from 100% organic earth friendly high powered cleansing oils.

These oils are great for the skin, the hair follicles, the earth, and the water, and some of them can even be individually ingested, (but of course not all of them).

This amazing multi-purpose soap that I recommend

everyone to start using is called "Dr. Bronner's Magic Soap." You can find it at most local health food stores and you can order it online. It is the best soap I have found on the market and I recommend you use it in place of any and all other soaps, shampoos, conditioners, and detergents.

As for toothpaste, when you use the most common toothpastes that you buy from the store with beautifully designed packaging that tricks you into thinking it is healthy, you also ingest a lot of chemicals through the glands in the mouth, including harmful and poisonous fluoride.

I always shop for natural mineral and oil based fluoride-free toothpastes to help avoid putting chemicals in my body. The toothpaste I like the most is made by "Tom's Toothpastes." It's a toothpaste that tastes good, is chemical free, and helps your mouth and body stay clean.

The unfortunate fact is that most of the water we use from our taps, shower heads, and sinks is entirely polluted with harmful chemicals, so the best water to put into your body is fresh spring water, which does not include harmful elements, toxins, chlorine, drugs, medication, metals, and fluoride found in most tap water today, plus it is filled with minerals (electrolytes) that help your body stay young, healthy, and well-balanced.

Water filters will help, but they won't get rid of all the chlorine, fluoride, and heavy metals from the tap water. The best thing to do is find a place where you can get fresh spring water that doesn't have any chemicals, and is full of the natural minerals that are so good for the body. A great resource that helped me find our local spring water is www.findaspring.com.

Chapter 4. So What About Meat?

I grew up on meat. Living in Montana for 18 years I can tell you that meat was not a delicacy, it was a necessity. Montanans swear by meat, and we eat every kind of meat possible. I've eaten deer, elk, bison, rabbit, moose, cow, sheep, pig, goat, chicken, and venison. Of course considering the water animals as well, I've eaten trout, salmon, halibut, shrimp, crab, crawdads, perch, bass, eel, oysters, and lobster.

I spent the first 18 years of my life on a meat and potato diet. Although I didn't think anything of it then, my entire outlook about eating meat and harming animals has been transformed due to the contemplation of the purpose of animals on the planet.

It wasn't until I did my very first five day cleanse in 2007, that all of the sudden meat started becoming less and less appealing to me. A few years prior, I had already stopped hunting and fishing; it just didn't feel right for me to kill animals anymore.

Then after I started cleansing my mind and body, I began to realize that meat is actually very unhealthy for you. I know it goes entirely against what we are taught in school - you remember the whole food pyramid, right?

In the food pyramid, meat was one of the biggest portions, along with dairy and carbohydrates that are recommended for us to eat, but at the same time, you have to understand that it was created by the USDA, (the United State Department of Agriculture,) and they have a vested interest in making sure that the sell of crops and livestock remain well balanced.

Unfortunately the food pyramid is wrong, including their new version of the pyramid, and following it has helped generate millions of obese children who would later join the tens of millions of adults who get dis-eases such as diabetes, arthritis, and cancer, unless their eating habits are changed permanently.

The education of eating the right foods start in the home and in school, and unfortunately the United States schools have one of the worst and most unhealthy sugar filled and processed diets in the entire world. Most of the foods the children eat are filled with killers like high fructose corn syrup, additives, pesticides, herbicides, unnatural sweeteners, cooked meat, MSG, and more! Unless we put an end to this, starting in our own homes, this trend will only continue to get worse.

So why not meat? Why is it unhealthy to eat? Well it's actually very simple to understand. Living beings, like ourselves, require living foods. It's not just the fact that it's MEAT that poses a problem for our bodies, it's COOKED MEAT! As soon as you cook anything, it dies.

Once you kill a cow or a sheep or a goat, and you begin to cook it, you transform the living tissues into dead tissues.

If you were to eat meat raw, in terms of your body receiving and utilizing the nutrients, it would almost be better for you then cooking it. Unfortunately with all of the hormones and additives we are giving the animals these days, not to mention the bacteria infestation that goes along with rotting flesh, you would probably die from the raw meat if you ate it.

If we are supposed to be like tigers and sharks and wolves, then why do we spend so much money and time hiding the disgusting flavor of it by marinating it and cooking it and salting and flavoring it, while the true carnivores on the planet salivate over rotten, stinky, bloody carcasses?

Well for one, it tastes good, right? I used to think so, but it's just like eating fast food. Have you ever stopped eating fast food for 6 months or a year, and then one day you went and ate a huge, greasy, cooked burger? If you have, I can tell you from experience, it probably made you sick to your stomach. That's an important point to understand.

Our bodies get accustomed to the food sources we put into them. While we may never become immune to the dis-eases caused by poisons, toxins, and cooked meat, we can adapt to them. While this adaptation may seem like a normal process, it can actually be quite dangerous.

The proof in this can be found by looking at our own experiences. Ask yourself this question, "how do I feel

when I eat a huge calorie filled greasy fast-food meal?"
At first, you might feel good, but then how do you feel
shortly thereafter? Your energy gets drained, your mind
gets weak, you fill a little tired or lazy, and you might ever
get heartburn or indigestion.

Those are all signs that the food or substance you just
put into your body is the wrong thing for you, though
when you eat food that is designed by the creator for all
human beings to benefit from, you always feel an
increase in energy, mental stamina, and vitality.

The reality is that vegetables, seeds and legumes, often
have more nutrients overall than a dead cooked animal,
but they have tons of amino acids and protein our bodies
need to live healthy long lives as well.

Here's an interesting fact to consider. When you look at
an animal like a coyote or a wolf who's diet is based
primarily on meat, you will notice that everything about
them is designed to be able to eat meat.

Their jaws are more pointed so it's easier to attack and
eat their prey. They have lot's of sharp canine teeth for

tearing the meat. They are fast and agile so they can chase down their prey.   They have special enzymes in their body so they don't get sick from the bacteria of rotting meat. They have a small digestive system that processes the meat quickly. And they are actually attracted to, and love the smell of, dead rotting flesh.

Not only that, but true carnivores and omnivores eat the entire animal; including the intestines filled with fecal matter – and they love it!

Now humans on the other hand have a rounded jaw like herbivores which is better for chewing grains, fruits, and vegetables. Humans only have a couple small canine teeth that can be used to tear into apples and similar foods. Humans have a larger digestive system which has a very hard time processing meat. Humans don't like the smell or taste of raw meat and rotting flesh, so they cook it.

If we analyze our designs as human beings, we're not even well equipped enough to eat meat, so we had to invent forks, knives, bbqs, and a whole industry of cooking gadgets, just so we can eat dead meat that has been proven to destroy the living cells in our bodies.

Can you imagine pulling a living fish out of the river and taking a big chomp into it's scaly, slimy flesh? How would that taste? How would it smell? Terrible, right? Well what makes it any different by cooking it? It doesn't make it any more humane or healthy to avoid catching the fish or killing the cow by going to the market and buying the meat that's already prepared. Do you have to cook and add seasoning to a banana, or an orange, or celery, or cucumber, or lettuce to make it have flavor? Absolutely not.

It seems to me that someone, or a group of someone's, have been fooling all of us into believing that it's OK for us to eat meat. Well now's the time to take back our consciousness and determine just for ourselves if it's really good to eat meat or not.

What I've discovered by quitting eating meat and eating a lot more fresh, raw, fruits, vegetables, nuts, grains, legumes, seeds and berries, is that I have more energy, more vitality, and a higher chance of living longer without dis-ease.

If you want a healthy, long living, vital body you should consider stopping eating cooked meat, especially cow, pig, and chicken, and start eating more whole foods that grow naturally all by itself just as the creator designed it for us. The best food for our bodies are diverse whole plant foods.

Can you imagine what your body feels like as it is constantly trying to process dead unhealthy food as it gets stuck in the intestines and colon?

The easiest, healthiest, and most beneficial foods for our bodies are outlined all throughout this document. You will find them in different sources, raw and cooked, and in different recipes, that are delicious, energizing, and much better for your mind, body, and spirit than any animal flesh could ever be.

Take the leap of faith with me and at least, for the two weeks that this cleanse goes for, do without any meat or dairy, and at the end of the two weeks you decide at that point if meat is a necessary element you want to keep in your diet.

I assure you that by the time you finish this first cleanse, you will feel more in tune with what your body really NEEDS, and you will be able to discern which types of foods make you feel good, and which types make you feel bad.

And if you want to eat meat after that, go ahead, nobody is stopping you.

Chapter 5. The Digestive Tract

I have been a huge fan of milk and cheese my entire life. I remember when my mom would grate the cheese for homemade tacos - I used to sneak in the kitchen, distract her, and as soon as she turned away, I would snatch handful after handful of the freshly grated salty orange sharp cheddar cheese.

Even though I have enjoyed cheese and milk for many years, it's unfortunate that most dairy products available in stores today are extremely harmful to the human body.

After nearly twenty years of drinking 1/4 gallon of milk per day, I finally stopped drinking it. I found a much better substitute. I drink organic soy milk and almond milk, which I often make at home easily, that is not created by GMO soy beans, and not only does it taste great, but I feel great as well.

Dairy is another one of those interesting and tricky food sources similar to meat. If you were to really analyze what you are eating or drinking, you will come to see that you have taken a healthy and nutritious substance, and killed and transformed every living nutrient in it, then put it into your body. That's what happens when they pasteurize and homogenize the milk. They cook it and kill it leaving nothing but a white pus-like substance that can do more harm than good.

Milk can be nutritious and healthy, but only when it's raw. Would a woman pump the milk out of her breast for her baby, then homogenize and pasteurize it before feeding it to the baby? Of course not! The baby needs the milk fresh and RAW with all of the living nutrients.

So if the mother and the baby both need fresh, RAW, uncooked, un-pasteurized, and un-homogenized milk, wouldn't it make sense for everyone to need it as well? I don't drink raw cow's milk anymore, but if you are going to drink any milk at all, it should be raw from a local farmer, otherwise I recommend eliminating all dairy from your diet.

But of course you only want to drink raw milk that comes from a cow or a goat who has been fed organic food and who has been treated with pure love by the owners. If a cow is experiencing bad feelings due to poor treatment, they will actually secrete harmful toxins into the milk, and your body will receive the after effects.

The same goes for cheese. Most cheese on the market is made from cooked milk that comes from cows who have been treated poorly, so all of the nutrients go right out the window. But even worse than that, cheese is a very sticky compound, and when it's ingested, it's very hard for your body to digest.

Cheese can be very binding and cause constipation in some people.

And if your intestine is blocked by this sticky cheese, even though you're eating and drinking healthy, your body may have trouble processing many of the nutrients you're taking in. This could very well be an explanation for many so called "healthy people" getting extremely sick, and even dying.

If you are going to continue eating cheese, then at the very least I would recommend you only eat small amounts and get the cheese that is made from RAW ORGANIC milk.

Most commercial brands of milk are pasteurized and homogenized and when they say you are getting calcium or Vitamin D, you have to remember that those statements are related to BEFORE they cook the milk. Once they cook it, the cheese changes.

I have liked eating cheese for many years, but I've decided to cut it out completely. Again, be careful with eating cheese and drinking homogenized or pasteurized milk because you want your body to be able to process as many nutrients as possible so you will stay healthy, happy, and live a long life!

Chapter 6. Cleansing the Liver and Gallbladder

All of the organs in the human body are important, but two of the hardest working and most important organs sit side by side like high-school buddies; Lenny the Liver and Georgie the Gall Bladder.

These two guys work extra hard every day trying to cleanse out all of the toxins you put into your body through soaps, water, foods, air, and liquids. Lenny the Liver produces bile and tosses it over to Georgie the Gall Bladder. Once Georgie receives the bile it stores it to help aid the digestion of fats that come from the food you eat. Every time you eat certain foods, Georgie spits out a little bile and sends it to Lenny to help break down the food during the digestion process.

This bile that is created also helps dissolve cholesterol. Cholesterol is a normal component of all living animals, the problem is when you take in excess cholesterol such as when eating cooked meat, it will eventually create heart dis-ease. What happens is that the liver secretes

cholesterol and it binds with the bile. If there is more
cholesterol than the bile can dissolve, it gets stored in the
gallbladder. Over time, this bile and cholesterol get
together and create gallstones.

It has been said that most human beings in the world
have some form of cholesterol gallstones. I didn't believe
it until I did this cleanse, and the proof came in hundreds
of small greenish colored hard floating balls. These
small gallstones usually don't pose a problem, that is unti
they get larger and create gallbladder problems, which
results in a lot of pain and discomfort.

As well, many of these gallstones are filled with bacteria,
and even though you may be full of nutrients and
seemingly healthy, these little stones stay lodged and
hidden away in your gallbladder secreting little bacteria
throughout your body day after day.

The way to avoid all of this is simply to cleanse the liver
and gallbladder a couple times per year, and try to avoid
eating cooked meats. Once you do the liver cleanse you
will be amazed at how many little stones come flowing
out of your gallbladder and into the toilet.

The liver cleanse that you will do is a very simple, yet amazing one. I tried it after being recommended by my older brother Joshua, and low and behold it really worked! The cleanse that I refer to was created by Dr. Hulda, and was created as a way to heal people of allergies and cancer. She says that allergies start in the liver and can be cured by simply cleansing it on a regular basis.

There are some skeptics who believe that the stones that come out are not gallstones but that they are composed of the lemon juice and olive oil that you take in; though the cleanse we do does not include any lemon juice, and the stones that came out were definitely the ones that are seen in pictures of cholesterol gallstones.

After doing the cleanse twice before writing this, as well as administering others through it as well, I have seen that this cleanse really works, and once you have the chance to try it you will be able to see if you have stones sitting inside your gallbladder just waiting to come out.

Chapter 7. Three Household Necessities

I have found that there are three major health items needed in every household, and they all come from a very well known healthy company called, "Bragg."

The first one is Bragg ACV (Apple Cider Vinegar). The second one is Bragg Liquid Aminos, and the third one is Bragg Ginger and Sesame Dressing.

My wife and I have been drinking ACV Tea (1 tablespoon apple cider vinegar, 1 tablespoon honey, and one cup of hot water) diligently for a number of years.

It all started when I had a Kombucha factory in my kitchen and I had been experimenting with these healthy bacteria that are needed in the digestive system to create a well-balanced immune system and digestive tract.

My cupboards reeked with the vivacity of vinegar and I had pounds of extra Kombucha mothers waiting for their turn to reproduce, sitting in my refrigerator. It was fun to create and watch this colony of healthy bacteria grow and produce little living babies, all while feeding on the sugar in the tea and producing a health-giving tonic called; Kombucha.

Once I started drinking the Kombucha on a daily basis, my digestive problems at that time began going away. After years of digestion problems and bloating, it was like a miracle had suddenly happened. So I began farming the Kombucha and sharing it with others.

But one day it got out of control. I was like a small business owner who reached the limit of their business model but wasn't ready to grow and became overwhelmed with customers that weren't manageable, and so I did what some small business owners do in that situation and I threw all the bacteria away.

I was a little devastated that all that work had suddenly disappeared, but I was relieved at the same time. Kombucha is great to make on your own if you just want to drink it for you and your family. It's also great because you can share it with others. Just be aware that it reproduces quickly and that you can either give away the

mother SCOBYs, or just throw them out so you don't end
up with a laboratory like I did.
Somehow during my Kombucha journey, I got turned ont
Bragg Apple Cider Vinegar.

Apple Cider Vinegar was used by Hippocrates to treat his
patients of many types of illnesses. Apple Cider Vinega
has been stated by people around the globe to help cure
themselves of skin diseases, heart diseases, blood
diseases, ulcers, intestinal problems, cancers, and a lot
of other very devastating dis-eases.

This very potent and strong combination of fermented
apples packs a very powerful punch and can bring
ultimate health and vitality to your daily life.

It only takes one teaspoon mixed with some warm water
and honey, and you are on your way to feeling more
energized, healthy, and alive. Just make sure to use a
wooden spoon when serving the ACV as it contains
natural acids that are good for your body, but bad when
mixed with metals.

I've included my best Kombucha recipe as part of this cleanse, and whether you drink ACV or Kombucha, I believe you will see a lasting difference in your overall health.

Chapter 8. Juicers and Blenders

Does this cleanse require that you have a juicer and a blender? Yes. The truth is there are so many different types of juicers and blenders out there. Some are definitely better than others, but whatever you can afford is what I would suggest you buy.

I've used multiple types of juicers and have stuck with one I found at Costco. It's been reliable and has two types of speed settings for the different densities of fruits and vegetables.

The juicers with the high-speed motors will kill some of the nutrients, but the best part is you will receive gobs of nutrients from fruits and vegetables you might not otherwise eat and in an easily accessible form.

Costco also has a powerful blender that's a few hundred dollars, but it's been well worth it in our family. Again, whatever you can afford is what I recommend.

The reason juicers are so important to your health is because you get to place multiple servings of fruits and vegetables, especially ones you don't like to eat very often, and juice them all into a very soluble form, and soak up the nutrients into your body right away, while creating a very delicious drink.

The downside to the juicer is that it removes the pulp, so you're missing out on the beneficial fiber that helps regulate your bowel movement and slowly process the natural sugars through your organs.

That's where the blender comes into play. The blender allows you to mix life-giving fruits and vegetables together, add a little honey and soy milk, and you have a very tasty, filling, and healthy drink.

Of course, the ultimate goal is to eat raw organic fruits, vegetables, nuts, seeds, berries, beans, and legumes every single day in place of cooked vegetables and meats, but in the meantime, juicers and blenders are well worth the investment and a great way to improve your overall health and consciousness.

The beauty of The Panacea Cleanse is that it is a hybrid cleanse, meaning that during the entire course of the cleanse, you will get the fiber your body needs to help with digestion while assimilating sugars correctly, and you will also give your organs a break from digesting whole foods so they can repair themselves and be in better condition to receive and process the nutrients that come from the food you eat and drink.

We utilize both the blender and the juicer in this cleanse so you can ease into the cleanse without going from one extreme to the other. We do this by starting with blended drinks, then move to the juiced drinks, and on to the pure water/master cleanse, and back out the same way.

Chapter 9. Preparation

We're almost ready to begin the cleanse. Are you excited? I'm always excited when it comes to doing a new cleanse. The important key here is to follow the entire system and don't get out of the cleanse too early.

If you do have to quit the cleansing process early, for whatever reason, then don't come out of it and start eating heavy foods right away, especially not meats or greasy good. It's important that if you leave the cleanse early then you should skip to day #11 in the cleanse and come out of it by following the plan and only eating what's recommended.

It's possible, and I've seen it first hand, that if you are cleansing, and you come out of it to eat a large greasy meal, you could become sick to your stomach, and even hospitalized.

You have to remember that you are cleansing all of the toxins out of your body and creating an alkaline and healthy environment so your body can heal itself.

If you immediately start putting greasy, chemical filled, unhealthy food back into your system, your body will reject it and show you that it does not want it any more. This is a good sign for your body, and should be paid attention to very closely. So make sure that when you come out of the cleanse to only eat fresh raw fruits and vegetables and follow the plan herein.

Chapter 10. Making Kombucha

Chapter 10 is optional, but if you do decide that you want to make your own tasty and health-giving Kombucha to have when you come out of the cleanse, I've supplied my very own recipe below.

You can order your organic, raw SCOBY and starter kit from Ebay, and have it mailed to your front doorstep as I've done in the past. Just find someone who has been making the raw and organic Kombucha in a smoke-free environment, and who has received a lot of good reviews on their Ebay profile.

Kombucha – Start 1 gallon of Kombucha 3 days before the cleanse so when you come out of the cleanse you will be able to refill your body with good bacteria that was lost during the cleanse.

The first time I made Kombucha, I used a recipe I found online that seemed like it was reliable. It was short, simple and direct. I followed it step by step. And in the end, my batch of Kombucha tea was full of mold!

I knew it was mold, but I had to do a lot of research to make sure it wasn't just how the MAMA SCOBY was supposed to look. If you ever get mold in your Kombucha batches, throw it away and start over! You will know if you get mold because it will look blue or green, or even white, but it will look just like it does on bread or fruits.

Since that experience, I researched, researched and researched how to make Kombucha THE RIGHT WAY! And since that Kombucha experience, fortunately I never had a moldy batch again!
So here is the step-by-step Kombucha recipe I use, on how to make Kombucha the right way, so your next batch of Kombucha will flourish with life, flavor and health!

Kombucha checklist: This recipe makes one gallon of ORGANIC Kombucha!

1. Organic green tea – You can buy bulk organic green tea, or you can buy it pre-packaged – you will need at least 30 of the packets or about 4 ounces of the bulk tea. (I also buy large reusable

tea bags from ebay that work great for the bulk loose leaf tea, and are great for preserving the environment.)

2. One gallon-sized GLASS jar.
3. One gallon of spring water or filtered water.
4. 4. A bottle of white vinegar. – Just PLAIN old white vinegar does the trick!
5. Cup of organic sugar. – I've used different kinds of organic sugar, and they've all turned out good.
6. One big metal pot for the stove.
7. One super large organic Mama! – Or otherwise known as a SCOBY. (Or three-five small mothers will work for one gallon)

Step one – Boil one gallon of filtered water on the metal pot on your stove.

Step two – Once the water comes to a boil, pour in the cup of sugar, stir it around for about one minute, then turn it off.

Step three – Put in the 30 tea bags, or about 18 tablespoons of the loose leaf tea in a reusable tea bag.

Step four – Let the tea bags sit between 5-8 minutes, then take it out.

Step five – Let the tea sit a few hours until it cools to room temperature. It needs to be room temperature, so it doesn't kill the mama!

Step six – While the tea is cooling, now you can prep the big glass jar. Clean your hands with the white vinegar, wash out the inside of the glass jar with the white vinegar rinse it out real good, and leave the vinegar in the glass jar. DON'T rinse it out with water afterwards.

Step seven – Once the tea has cooled to room temperature, pour it into the glass jar.
Step eight – Rinse your hands with vinegar again, then grab the SCOBY mama with your bare hands, and insert it, PLUS THE K-TEA that came with it, into the glass jar.

Step nine – Cover the top of the glass jar with a SINGLE paper towel, and secure it with a rubber band.

Step ten – put it way up in the top of a cupboard where it won't be touched for the next 12-20 days.

Step eleven – If it's above 65 degrees in the cupboard, you will want to taste it at about the 10-15th day. If it's cooler, it will take a bit longer. You can taste it between the 15th – 20th day.

How to make Kombucha carbonation, fruits, and flavors.

Make sure never to add any flavors, fruits, flavored teas, or anything of the sort to the Kombucha while it is fermenting. It can cause it to kill the mama.

Carbonation

The best way to make your Kombucha have more of the natural carbonation is to do a second fermentation process.

After the Kombucha tea is ready, what to do is bottle it in glass jars. The best jars are glass jars with plastic lids. Then put them high up in the cupboard again for about 2-5 days. During that time the carbonation will form.

(NOTE: NEVER TOUCH THE KOMBUCHA TO METAL)
So no metal lids on the jars. Kombucha makes acetic acid, a good acid for digestion, but when it touches meta it makes the Kombucha acidic.

Fruits and Flavors

Once you have the final jars filled with Kombucha, and they've gone through the second fermentation process, now you're ready to add fruits and flavors. This part is fun and you can experiment with which fruits and flavors you like best. The best way is to get a juicer, and juice your own fruits and veggies, and then add about 10%-20% of the juice into the bottles with the Kombucha.

Once you've added the fruits and flavors, if you don't drink it right away, make sure to keep it in the fridge so it can last as long as possible. Drink and ENJOY!

Where to get a mama – SCOBY

You can get a scoby, or a mama from anybody else who has one. The important things to make sure is that they have been handled with care, they have always used organic and filtered ingredients, and that they don't smoke in the house and make sure they come with some starter K-TEA.

Another way you can start is to go to the health food store and buy 3 bottles of the original raw organic Kombucha from Synergy, and pour those into your tea mix and let it ferment. It will create a great batch of Kombucha.

Take care and enjoy!

My blog for more info about Kombucha –
For more info, visit: http://mybuchatea.wordpress.com/

DAY BEFORE THE CLEANSE

Weight: _________________

Stomach circumference:_________________

Headaches, Pain, Ailments, Dis-Eases, Stomach Problems etc…:

____

____

____

____

DAY 1

Weight: _______________

Stomach circumference:_________________

Headaches, Pain, Ailments, Dis-Eases, Stomach Problems, Overall Improvements etc…:

____

____

____

____

DAY 2

Weight: _______________

Stomach circumference:_______________

Headaches, Pain, Ailments, Dis-Eases, Stomach
Problems, Overall Improvements etc...:

____

____

____

____

DAY 3

Weight: _______________

Stomach circumference:_______________

Headaches, Pain, Ailments, Dis-Eases, Stomach
Problems, Overall Improvements etc...:

____

____

____

DAY 4

Weight: ________________

Stomach circumference:__________________

Headaches, Pain, Ailments, Dis-Eases, Stomach
Problems, Overall Improvements etc...:

____

____

____

____

DAY 5

Weight: ________________

Stomach circumference:__________________

Headaches, Pain, Ailments, Dis-Eases, Stomach
Problems, Overall Improvements etc...:

____

____

____

____

DAY 6

Weight: _________________

Stomach circumference:_________________

Headaches, Pain, Ailments, Dis-Eases, Stomach
Problems, Overall Improvements etc…:

____

____

____

____

DAY 7

Weight: _________________

Stomach circumference:_________________

Headaches, Pain, Ailments, Dis-Eases, Stomach
Problems, Overall Improvements etc…:

____

____

____

____

DAY 8

Weight: ___________________

Stomach circumference:___________________

Headaches, Pain, Ailments, Dis-Eases, Stomach
Problems, Overall Improvements etc…:

____

____

____

____

DAY 9

Weight: ___________________

Stomach circumference:___________________

Headaches, Pain, Ailments, Dis-Eases, Stomach
Problems, Overall Improvements etc…:

____

____

____

____

DAY 10

Weight: ______________

Stomach circumference:__________________

Headaches, Pain, Ailments, Dis-Eases, Stomach
Problems, Overall Improvements etc…:

____

____

____

____

DAY 11

Weight: ______________

Stomach circumference:__________________

Headaches, Pain, Ailments, Dis-Eases, Stomach
Problems, Overall Improvements etc…:

____

____

____

____

DAY 12

Weight: ______________

Stomach circumference:__________________

Headaches, Pain, Ailments, Dis-Eases, Stomach
Problems, Overall Improvements etc…:

____

____

____

____

DAY 13

Weight: ______________

Stomach circumference:__________________

Headaches, Pain, Ailments, Dis-Eases, Stomach
Problems, Overall Improvements etc…:

____

____

____

____

Chapter 12. The Cleanse

(Below is what we will cleanse over the next 12 days)

Days 1-2

Blended Drinks and Water Only

(Liver, kidneys.)

Days 3-4 – (Evening of Day 3 and Morning of Day 4 is the Liver and Gallbladder Cleanse)

Juiced Drinks, and Water Only

(Gallbladder, Heart, Skin, Hair, Nails, Bones)

Days 5-7

Master Cleanse, and Water Only

(Digestive System, Ascending and Descending Colon)

Days 8-9

Juiced Drinks, and Water Only

(Eyes, Brain, Skin, Immune System)

Days 10-11

Blended Drinks and Water Only

(Stomach, Muscles, Tendons, Ligaments, Liver, Kidneys)

Day 12

Recovery Meals - Healthy Eating Habits - Good Bacteria
Kombucha - ACV Tea and Honey

Days 13-16

Healthy eating recipes

Cost to do ORGANIC cleanse: Roughly $12.89 Per
Person Per Day

SUCCESS TIP: MAKE SURE TO GO TO USE THE
TRACKING CHART TO MEASURE YOUR WEIGHT,
SIZE, AND EXPERIENCE BEFORE, DURING, AND
AFTER THE CLEANSE.

12 Day Cleanse Shopping List

Produce:

- Fresh spinach leaves: 5 cups
- Fresh parsley: 60 leaves
- Large grapefruits: 4
- Large apples: 8
- Bananas: 15
- Dried cranberries: 6 tablespoons
- Large slices of ginger: 2 slices (size of a $1.00 coin)
- Large slices of tomatoes: 1 large tomato
- Florets of broccoli: 4 florets
- Large sticks of celery: 8 sticks
- Large bell peppers (orange or yellow): 1/2 large bell pepper
- Large watermelon: 1
- Fresh strawberries: 1 1/2 cups
- Fresh mint leaves: 2 1/4 cups
- Large leaves of kale: 6 leaves
- Large carrots: 36
- Small oranges: 21 small oranges (or 12 large)
- Lemons: 6
- Small pears: 3 medium-sized pears
- Small avocado: 3 small avocados
- Romaine lettuce: 16 large leaves
- Green chard: 1 regular bunch
- Onion: 1/2 cup chopped onion
- Garlic: 2 teaspoons minced fresh garlic
- Roma tomatoes: 2 large tomatoes

Pantry Items:

- Raw millet or flax seeds: 3 1/4 cups
- Honey: 9 tablespoons (or add to taste)
- Organic soy milk or almond milk (optional): As needed
- Bee pollen (optional): As needed
- Organic grade B maple syrup: 3 cups (or adjust to taste)
- Cayenne pepper: 2 1/4 teaspoons (or add more to taste)
- Sea salt: As needed
- Lentils: 1 cup
- Olive oil: 1 tablespoon

Beverages:

- Spring water: 240 ounces (or adjust based on daily needs)
- Kombucha or other probiotic supplement (e.g., Kefir or Kimchi): As needed

Miscellaneous:

- Epsom salt: 4 tablespoons
- Freshly juiced apple juice: 6 cups (for liver cleanse)

Please note that the quantities mentioned above are approximate and may vary based on personal preferences and serving sizes.

DAY 1 - Blended Drinks + Water Only

(Liver, kidneys)

BREAKFAST AND SNACKS

Morning Super Tonic

Recipe makes about 48 ounces. Can drink as much as desired throughout the day.

- 1 cup fresh spinach leaves
- 15 leaves fresh parsley
- 1 large grapefruit - cut into 4 pieces with pith and skin taken off
- 5 heaping tablespoons (1/3 Cup) raw millet or flax seed
- 1 banana
- 40 ounces spring water
- 3 tablespoons honey or add to taste

- OPTIONAL - Use organic soy milk or almond milk in place of water for protein and more flavor. Add 1 tablespoon of bee pollen for additional amino acids)

Blend all ingredients together and enjoy.

LUNCH AND DINNER

Liver Bliss

Recipe Makes About 48 Ounces. Can drink as much as desired during the day and evening.

- 2 tablespoons dried cranberries
- 4 heaping tablespoons raw millet
- 1 large slice of ginger (size of a $1.00 coin)
- 1 large apple - cut into 4 pieces
- 1 cup fresh spinach leaves
- 1 banana
- 15 leaves fresh parsley
- 3 tablespoons honey or add to taste

- OPTIONAL - Use organic soy milk or almond milk in place of water for protein and more flavor. Add 1 tablespoon of bee pollen for additional amino acids)

Blend all ingredients together and enjoy.

NOTE: You can also squeeze fresh lemon or lime into a glass of spring water and drink to help overcome any hunger pangs or gas buildup throughout the day.

DAY 2 - Blended Drinks + Water Only

(Liver, kidneys)

BREAKFAST AND SNACKS

Morning Super Tonic

Recipe makes about 48 ounces. Can drink as much as desired throughout the day.

• 1 cup fresh spinach leaves

• 15 leaves fresh parsley

• 1 large grapefruit - cut into 4 pieces with pith and skin taken off

• 5 heaping tablespoons (1/3 Cup) raw millet or flax seed

• 1 banana

• 40 ounces spring water

• 3 tablespoons honey or add to taste

- OPTIONAL - Use organic soy milk or almond milk in place of water for protein and more flavor. Add 1 tablespoon of bee pollen for additional amino acids)

Blend all ingredients together and enjoy.

LUNCH AND DINNER

Livin' Grape Goodness

Recipe makes about 48 ounces. Can drink as much as desired throughout the day and evening.

- 1 cup fresh grapes
- 2 tablespoons dried cranberries
- 1 cup fresh spinach leaves
- 1 large apple - Cut into 4 Slices
- 15 leaves fresh parsley
- 5 heaping tablespoons (1/3 Cup) raw millet or flax seed
- 1 banana
- 40 ounces spring water
- 3 tablespoons honey or add to taste

- OPTIONAL - Use organic soy milk or almond milk in place of water for protein and more flavor. Add 1 tablespoon of bee pollen for additional amino acids)
Blend all ingredients together and enjoy.

DAY 3 - Juiced Drinks + Liver Cleanse

(Gallbladder, Heart, Skin, Hair, Nails, Bones)

BREAKFAST

The Champion's Breakfast

- 6 large carrots
- 2 large apples
- 7 small oranges (Or 4 large)
- 1 large grapefruit
- 2 large leaves of kale (Stems Removed)

Push everything through juicer and enjoy!

LUNCH AND SNACKS

Waterberry Fresca.

- 1 large watermelon – remove green outer skin, keep inner white pith intact for juicing
- ¾ cup fresh strawberries
- ¾ cup fresh mint leaves

Push everything through juicer and enjoy!

DINNER

Cold Stomper

- 1 large tomato
- 2 florets of broccoli
- 4 large carrots
- 2 large sticks of celery
- 1 inch size piece garlic
- ½ large bell pepper (orange or yellow)

Push everything through juicer and enjoy!

(You will want to finish drinking this by 5:30pm since you will take your first gallbladder drink at 6:00pm)

DAY 3 – EVENING, GALLBLADDER AND LIVER CLEANSE (Start preparing at 4:00pm on Day 3)

LIVER CLEANSE RECIPE

(Best done on a night where you don't have to work the next day so you can rest and relax if needed)

- ½ cup olive oil - extra virgin cold pressed

- 1 large grapefruit
- 4 tablespoons of Epsom Salt
- 1 ½ cups water and 1 ½ cups fresh apple juice - about
  5 large apples

PLEASE READ BELOW BEFORE DOING GALLBLADDER AND LIVER CLEANSE

The Gallbladder flush is a powerful cleanse I first found out about through Dr. Hulda. Dr. Hulda states that she has conducted over 1000 of these cleanses without a single bad result . Some people say this flush can be harmful because of the amount of Epsom Salt you take. The amount of Salt Dr. Hulda recommends is a lot of salt and though the first time I did the cleanse I didn't have any problems, the second time I did it I felt a little queasy and couldn't finish all of the salt.

Though I didn't finish all of the salt drink the second time I did the cleanse, both times I had great results in passing stones. I passed over 100 gallstones the first time, and over 70 gallstones the second time. These gallstones build up in the gallbladder because of the bile that is produced by the liver to help digest food.

What happens is that the bilary tubing that the bile goes through to get to the intestines gets filled up with excess balls of bile, known as gallstones. These gallstones are basically made up of bile, water, cholesterol, and bile Salt.

Due to their porous nature, they easily attract bacteria and parasites, making it nearly impossible to get fully healthy or overcome dis-ease if these little stones are in your body. The number one cause of gallstones is failure of the liver to dump out bile correctly.   I have read that nearly 80% of people have these little gallstones without even knowing it.

The only time you know that you have gallstones is by either waiting until you become extremely ill and possibly dying, or by flushing them out by doing a gallbladder cleanse like this one.

The great thing about this flush is that it not only cleanses out your gallbladder and helps get rid of these stones, but it also cleanses out your liver at the same time.

Both my wife and myself did this cleanse, getting rid of stones. Once they come out, they look like little green, black, red, or yellowish hard balls and can be as small as a grain of sand or as large as a golf ball. Though if you are not experiencing any symptoms of gallbladder disease, it is most likely that yours will range from the size of sand to the size of small pebbles. My wife only had about thirty of them and they were all smaller than a little pebble, while both times many of mine were as big as ½ inch across.

There was no pain when passing these stones because of the type of recipe that is used to get them out. The olive oil helps them pass easily and the Epsom Salt opens everything up so they come out.

There is a heed of warning when doing this flush, and that is to know if your body can handle the Epsom Salt or not. The recipe calls for a lot of Epsom Salt and usually causes some nausea. If at any time you feel sick or that you cannot continue with the flush, make sure to drink a large glass of water and contact your physician if needed.

Because of the large amount of Epsom salt Dr. Hulda's recipe calls for, and the fact that both my wife and I weren't able to finish all the salt the second time around and still passed plenty of stones, we have reduced the recipe to 2 Tablespoons of Epsom Salt to help prevent nausea when drinking the salt.

So listen to your body. Don't push yourself too far past your threshold, and make sure to drink lots of water. The drinks are strong, and challenging to take down, though after the flush is completed, which is only about 12 hours it is a great feeling to have known that you got all that bacteria and cholesterol buildup out of your body.

If you have any questions about this portion of the cleanse which aren't answered here, please refer to the FAQs on page 11.

So if you're ready, here's the process. Try to follow it exact as the timeline suggests on the following pages. You can move the time to fit your schedule, just make sure to move each hour ahead or behind as needed.

LIVER CLEANSE PROCESS

4:00 PM or So...

Get your Epsom Salt ready. Mix 2 tablespoons into 3 cups of fresh juiced apple juice inside a large glass or mason jar.

This makes FOUR servings, 3/4 cup each. Set the jar in the refrigerator to get ice cold (this is for convenience and taste only).

6:00 P.M. – 1st Serving

Pull the mixture out of the fridge, stir up and drink **one serving** (3/4 cup) of the mixture. You may also drink a few mouthfuls of water or organic fresh squeezed juice afterwards to rinse your mouth.

8:00 P.M. – 2nd Serving

Repeat by drinking **another 3/4 cup serving** of the Epsom salt mixture. Get your regular nighttime chores done. The timing is pretty important for success; try not to be more than 15 minutes early or late.

9:45 P.M. – Prepare Olive Oil Mixture....

Pour 1/2 cup expeller pressed olive oil into a separate glass or mason jar. Squeeze 1 large grapefruit by hand into a measuring cup. Remove pulp. You should have at least 1/2 cup of grapefruit juice. Add this to the olive oil. Close the jar tightly with the lid and mix or shake hard until watery.

Now visit the bathroom once or more even it makes you late for your ten o'clock drink. Try not to be more than 15 minutes late.

10:00 PM. – Drink Olive Oil Mixture

Drink the Olive Oil mixture you have mixed. If you normally have trouble sleeping you can take 4 ornithine capsules with the first sips to make sure you will sleep through the night, or three melatonin tablets.

Try to drink the olive oil mixture within 5 minutes. It will be strong and hard to take down, but it's easiest to do it all in one shot.

Lie down on your back right away. You might fail to get some stones out if you don't. The sooner you lie down the more stones you can get out. Try to be ready for bed ahead of time. As soon as the drink is down walk to your bed and lie down flat on your back with your head up on the pillow.

Put your mind into focus on cleansing your liver. Try to keep perfectly still for at least 20 minutes. You might feel a set of stones traveling along the bile ducts like little balls. There is no pain because the bile duct valves are open (thanks to the Epsom Salt). Now go to sleep.

Next morning upon awakening

6:00 A.M. or so – 3rd Serving

Upon awakening take your **third serving of Epsom Salt.** If you have indigestion or nausea wait until it is gone before drinking the Epsom Salt. Try to go to the restroom and have a bowel movement, it will help with any nausea. If you feel nausea upon awakening, drink a large glass of water and see how you feel. If you feel better after 15 minutes, you may continue with the third glass of Salt mixture, if you do not feel better and you continue to feel worse, you may consider calling your physician. I found that with the third dose, you can get rid of up to 70 stones or more. You may go back to bed. Try not to take this third drink before 6:00 AM

2 hours later – 8:00 A.M. or so – 4th Serving

If you feel ok, take your **fourth (the last) serving** of Epsom Salt mixture. Drink 3/4 cups of the mixture. You may go back to bed. If you do not feel well enough, drink a large glass of water and wait 15 minutes to see if you feel better. You can still pass stones even without the fourth drink. To get the maximum results it is best to take the fourth drink, but only take it if you feel well enough.

After 2 more hours you may continue with 4th Day Cleansing Plan.

How well did you do? Check the toilet for any small, greenish marble looking stones. Gallstones float because of the cholesterol inside. You can have up to 100 or more. Some might be bigger than others.

DAY 4 - Juiced Drinks + Water

(Gallbladder, Heart, Skin, Hair, Nails, Bones)

BREAKFAST

The Champion's Breakfast

- 6 large carrots
- 2 large apples
- 7 small oranges (Or 4 large)
- 1 large grapefruit
- 2 large leaves of kale (Stems Removed)

Push everything through juicer and enjoy!

LUNCH AND SNACKS

Waterberry Fresca.

- 1 large watermelon – remove green outer skin, keep inner white pith intact for juicing
- ¾ cup fresh strawberries
- ¾ cup fresh mint leaves

Push everything through juicer and enjoy!

DINNER

Cold Stomper

- 1 large tomato

- 2 florets of broccoli

- 4 large carrots

- 2 large sticks of celery

- 1 inch size piece garlic

- ½ large bell pepper (orange or yellow)

Push everything through juicer and enjoy!

DAYS 5-7 – Master Cleanse + Water

(Digestive System, Ascending and Descending Colon)

BREAKFAST, LUNCH, SNACKS, AND DINNER

The master cleanse was first written about and studied by Stanley Burroughs. Having done the master cleanse multiple times, and having administered others through it as well, I have come to realize that by preparing for it days in advance as we have done here, the results are much more effective than otherwise.

For the next three days you will only drink the master cleanse recipe as well as additional glasses of pure spring water. At this point we have supplied all the major organs with a tremendous amount of vitamins, nutrients, minerals, amino acids, and beneficial enzymes in liquid format to help the body get used to a liquid diet as well as help combat the free radicals that are floating around damaging the cells.

Now during this portion of the cleanse you will be ready

to cleanse out all of the toxins that are residing within your cells. During these next three days you will allow your digestive organs to take a rest, potentially for the first time in their entire lives, and begin the initial phase of their rejuvenation process. You will also be cleansing out any toxins and buildup that have been residing within the colon and digestive tract, allowing your body to be clean and receptive to the nutrients you will be packing on after these next three days.

MASTER CLEANSE RECIPE

(Per 8 ounces of room temperature filtered water)
- 2 tablespoons of fresh lemon juice (approx. 1/2 large lemon squeezed or juiced without peel
- 2 tablespoons organic grade B maple syrup. Not maple flavored sugar syrup. You want pure maple syrup. Grade A will work as well.
- 1/10 teaspoon cayenne pepper or add more to taste

Per gallon - a gallon can last a half day, full day or a day and a half depending on how much you drink
- 1.5 Teaspoons Cayenne Pepper Per Gallon
- Original recipe calls for 2 cups of Fresh Lemon Juice

Per Gallon

• Original recipe calls for 2 cups of Organic Grade B Maple Syrup Per Gallon

(I only use 1 to 1.5 cups of lemon and 1 to 1.5 cups maple syrup depending on how sweet and sour I want it)   But I like to add 3 large teaspoons of cayenne

(Here's a Simple Measuring Resource)
128 Ounces in a gallon
1TBSP = .5 Ounce

The easiest thing to do is buy three gallons of spring water from your local grocery store in single gallons and pour out ¼ of the gallon into a glass or pitcher you can drink later.

In the rest of the ¾ gallon of spring water in the container you purchased, you wll add the fresh squeezed lemon juice, maple syrup, and cayenne pepper. These ingredients together help cleanse, detoxify, energize, and keep your hunger pangs relatively unnoticed.

If you feel hungry at all, simply take a drink of the master cleanse and you will feel fine. It is important at this stage of the cleanse to note that if you need to stop the cleanse for any reason, you absolutely should not break your cleanse by eating meat, bacon, greasy foods, processed foods, or any fast food. Your body has been purifying itself and if you stop the cleanse and start putting toxins back into it right away, you could become seriously ill.

If you have to stop the cleanse, skip to Day 11 in the cleanse and finish it from there, otherwise continue on like normal for the next three days with the Master Cleanse. The three days will pass quickly and you will feel great afterwards so I encourage you to continue on and finish through until the end. You will thank yourself for doing so.

DAY 8 - Juiced Drinks + Water

(Brain, Eyes, Skin, Immune System)

BREAKFAST

The Champion's Breakfast

- 6 large carrots
- 2 large apples
- 7 small oranges (Or 4 large)
- 1 large grapefruit
- 2 large leaves of kale (Stems Removed)

Push everything through juicer and enjoy!

LUNCH AND SNACKS

Blue Waterberry Fresca.

(Makes about 1 Gallon, Drink throughout entire day)

- 1 large watermelon
- 1 cup of blueberries
- ¾ cup fresh mint leaves

Push everything through juicer and enjoy!

DINNER

Cold Stomper

- 1 large tomato

- 2 florets of broccoli

- 4 large carrots

- 2 large sticks of celery

- 1 inch size piece garlic

- ½ large bell pepper (orange or yellow)

Push everything through juicer and enjoy!

DAY 9 - Juiced Drinks + Water

(Brain, Eyes, Skin, Immune System)

BREAKFAST

The Champion's Breakfast

- 6 large carrots
- 2 large apples
- 7 small oranges (Or 4 large)
- 1 large grapefruit
- 2 large leaves of kale (Stems Removed)

Push everything through juicer and enjoy!

LUNCH AND SNACKS

Blue Waterberry Fresca.

(Makes about 1 Gallon, Drink throughout entire day)

- 1 large watermelon
- 1 cup of blueberries
- ¾ cup fresh mint leaves

Push everything through juicer and enjoy!

DINNER

Cold Stomper

- 1 large tomato

- 2 florets of broccoli

- 4 large carrots

- 2 large sticks of celery

- 1 inch size piece garlic

- ½ large bell pepper (orange or yellow)

Push everything through juicer and enjoy!

DAY 10 – Blended Drinks + Water

(Liver, kidneys)

BREAKFAST AND SNACKS

Morning Super Tonic

Recipe makes about 48 ounces. Can drink as much as desired throughout the day.

- 1 cup fresh spinach leaves
- 15 leaves fresh parsley
- 1 large grapefruit - cut into 4 pieces with pith and skin taken off
- 5 heaping tablespoons (1/3 Cup) raw millet or flax seed
- 1 banana
- 40 ounces spring water
- 3 tablespoons honey or add to taste

- OPTIONAL - Use organic soy milk or almond milk in place of water for protein and more flavor. Add 1 tablespoon of bee pollen for additional amino acids)

Blend all ingredients together and enjoy.

LUNCH AND DINNER

Fiber and Protein Bananza

• 2 tablespoons dried cranberries

• 1 cup raw grapes

• 1/3 cup raw millet

• 1 large apple - Cut into 4 pieces

• 1 cup fresh spinach leaves

• 1 banana

• ¾ cup raw nuts - Can be any mixture of almonds, cashews, peanuts, sunflower seeds, brazilian nuts, pepitas, or any other raw nuts or seeds

• 40 ounces spring water

• 3 tablespoons honey or add to taste

- OPTIONAL - Use organic soy milk or almond milk in place of water for protein and more flavor. Add 1 tablespoon of bee pollen for additional amino acids)

Blend all ingredients together and enjoy.

DAY 11 – Blended Drinks + Water

BREAKFAST AND SNACKS

Morning Super Tonic

Recipe makes about 48 ounces. Can drink as much as desired throughout the day.

- 1 cup fresh spinach leaves
- 15 leaves fresh parsley
- 1 large grapefruit - cut into 4 pieces with pith and skin taken off
- 5 heaping tablespoons (1/3 Cup) raw millet or flax seed
- 1 banana
- 40 ounces spring water
- 3 tablespoons honey or add to taste

- OPTIONAL - Use organic soy milk or almond milk in place of water for protein and more flavor. Add 1 tablespoon of bee pollen for additional amino acids)

Blend all ingredients together and enjoy.

LUNCH AND DINNER

Fiber and Protein Bananza

- 2 tablespoons dried cranberries
- 1 cup raw grapes
- 1/3 cup raw millet
- 1 large apple - Cut into 4 pieces
- 1 cup fresh spinach leaves
- 1 banana
- ¾ cup raw nuts - Can be any mixture of almonds, cashews, peanuts, sunflower seeds, brazilian nuts, pepitas, or any other raw nuts or seeds
- 40 ounces spring water
- 3 tablespoons honey or add to taste

- OPTIONAL - Use organic soy milk or almond milk in place of water for protein and more flavor. Add 1 tablespoon of bee pollen for additional amino acids)

Blend all ingredients together and enjoy.

DAY 12 – REBUILD. EAT GOOD. FEEL GOOD.

It's time to start eating raw whole foods again and rejuvenate the cells

BREAKFAST

- 1 banana
- 1 orange
- 1/2 grapefruit
- 1/2 apple

(Cut banana, orange, grapefruit, and apple into bite size pieces and eat piece by piece)

- Drink 1 glass of fresh squeezed carrot juice - 6-8 large carrots pushed through the juicer
- 1 glass of spring water

LUNCH

Sweet and Sour Salad

- 4 large leaves romaine lettuce
- 1 cup fresh spinach leaves
- 1 medium ripened pear – diced into small 1" chunks
- 1 small avocado – diced into small 1" slices

-Dressing

• 1 tablespoon of fresh lemon juice squeezed from lemo

Mix lettuce and spinach together in a bowl, then add pea
and avocado and mix lightly with greens, sprinkle
dressing over salad, and add a dash of sea salt. Enjoy!

• Drink 16 ounces of your homemade or store bought
Kombucha or other probiotic supplement such as Kefir o
Kimchi to refill your healthy microflora bacteria.

DAILY SNACKS

• 2-3 raw whole carrots
• A couple handfuls or more of raw nuts and seeds
• Any combination of fresh fruit and vegetable juices

DINNER

1 Bowl of Veggie Lentil Soup

Recipe makes about 4 bowls

• 8 cups water
• 1 cup lentils
• 1 Tbs olive oil
• ½ cup chopped onion
• 1 tsp minced fresh garlic
• 1 Lg roma tomato

- 3 reg size roughly chopped carrots
- 2 reg size roughly chopped celery stalks
- 1reg bunch of green chard cut into bite size
- sea salt and pepper to taste

In a large pot bring the water to boil. Add the lentils, bring to boil, put the lid on and lower to medium-low heat and simmer until lentils are al dente (15 minutes or so).

While the lentils cook, heat the oil in a medium skillet over medium-low heat. Add the onion and garlic and sauté for 3-5 minutes then add the tomato and sauté until the it has become like a sauce.

Check the lentils. If they are al dente, add the "sauce", carrots, celery, chard, salt and pepper to the pot and simmer with lid on for 10-15 minutes more. Enjoy!

Chapter 13. The Follow Up Healthy Living Plan

CONGRAULATIONS, YOU COMPLETED THE
PANACEA CLEANSE!

It is a challenge and a journey to experience this cleanse
and only those who've gone through it and completed the
entire process can truly fill the sensations and
accomplishments that come with it. I commend you for
sticking with it till the end. If for any reason you weren't
able to make it all the way through, not to worry, give
yourself a couple of months, prepare your mind to
complete it until the end, and give it another go.

The follow up healthy living plan will take an entire book
to write about, and therefore keep an eye out for it as I
am already in the process of writing it by first practicing
living it in my own daily life.

In the meantime, please refer to the healthy eating bullet
points in terms of how to stabilize your diet and begin
eating as healthy and pure as possible. With the help of

my lovely wife, I've included some very simple, tasty, healthy recipes you can use for maintaining a healthy diet.

Healthy Eating Bullet Points:

• Add probiotic supplement to first the week after cleanse
• ACV + honey at least once per day
• Eat a full combination of organic fruits, vegetables, nuts, seeds, legumes, whole grains, and herbs as much as possible
• Eat raw as much as you can
• No meat, no dairy, no cheese, no alcohol, no smoking, no drugs (I know it sounds easier than it is, but it becomes easier and easier with practice)
• Small healthy portions of food, (not-overeating) multiple times per day with lots of fiber, vitamins, and minerals

If you follow the recommendations laid out in this book you will have begun a life transforming adventure and will be on the path to a pure lifestyle of health, happiness, and longevity.

The Panacea Cleanse should be conducted at least once

per year, if not more, to sustain long term health and vitality. If you have any comments, experiences, or successes you'd like to share, please email them to info@thepanaceacommunity. I'd love to hear from you.

DAYS 13 – 16 SHOPPING LIST

Produce:

- Medium carrots (18-20)
- Bananas
- Apples (9-10 medium)
- Spinach (2 handfuls)
- Lemon
- Kale leaves (6 large)
- Red cabbage (1 1/2 cups diced)
- Julienne carrots (1 1/2 cups)
- Pecans (1/2 cup)
- Pear
- Peppermint or herbal tea
- Celery stalks (4)
- Garlic cloves (2)
- Kaffir lime leaves (2)
- Baby bok choy
- Broccoli florets (1 1/4 cups)
- Cherry tomatoes (1 cup + 1/2 cup)
- Avocado (1 1/2 cups diced)
- Cilantro leaves
- Pineapple (about 1/2 cup roughly chopped)
- Cucumber
- Sweet potato (about 2-inch piece)
- Jicama (about 1/2 cup roughly chopped)

- Orange (1 large)
- Sweet corn kernels (1 1/4 cups)
- Diced red bell pepper (1/2 cup)
- Black olives (1 1/2 tablespoons sliced)
- Tomatoes (3 medium + 1/2 small)
- Basil leaves
- Dates (2)
- Oregano leaves
- Rosemary
- Watermelon (1/2 cup diced)
- Cantaloupe (1/2 cup)
- Orange bell pepper (1/2 cup julienne)
- Beets (1/2 cup julienne)
- Hemp seeds (1 tablespoon + 1 tablespoon)
- Romaine lettuce leaves (8)
- Dried cherries (2 tablespoons)
- Walnuts (1/4 cup)
- Grapes
- Mango (1/4 cup diced)
- Dried cranberries (2 tablespoons)
- Raw pepitas (2 tablespoons)
- Flax seeds (1 tablespoon)
- Black sesame seeds (1 tablespoon)
- Green chard
- Onion
- Roma tomato (2 medium)
- Carrots (6 medium)
- Celery stalks (4 medium)
- Lentils (1 cup)
- Green beans
- Zucchini
- Fresh ginger (1 slice, size of a US quarter)
- Green bell pepper (1)
- Fresh cilantro (for garnish)

Pantry/Other:

- Apple cider vinegar
- Honey
- Peanut butter
- Oregano tea or other herbal tea
- Kombucha (2 bottles)
- Raw sprouted bread (5 slices)
- Coconut oil
- Cold-pressed olive oil
- Sea salt
- Water
- Oats
- Cinnamon powder or cinnamon stick
- Almond milk
- Organic soy milk
- Honey (optional)
- Whole grain mix pizza crust
- Macadamia nuts (1/4 cup)
- Olive oil (1 teaspoon + 2 tablespoons)
- Lemon juice (1/2 tablespoon + 1/2 tablespoon)
- Sun-dried tomatoes (1 tablespoon)
- Fresh garlic
- Fresh lime
- Fresh cracked black pepper
- Almonds
- Apple cider vinegar (for salad dressing)
- Bragg Ginger and Sesame dressing

Please note that the quantities for some ingredients might not be specified in the recipes, so you can adjust them according to your preferences and serving sizes.

Chapter 14. Recipes for After The Cleanse

DAY 13

BREAKFAST

- 1 glass of water
- 1 glass of carrot juice: 8-10 medium carrots
- 1 banana with about 1/2 tsp peanut butter for each bite
- 1 cup ACV tea...
        -1 1/2 cups of warm water
        -1 Tbs Apple Cider Vinegar
        -1 Tbs honey
        - *Stir with wooden spoon and enjoy!*

SNACK

- 1 glass of water
- 1 apple or fruit of your choice
- 1 cup oregano tea or other herbal tea(add honey for flavor)
- 1 12oz glass of Kombucha

LUNCH

- 1 glass of water
- 1 glass of fresh juice: 4-5 medium apples + 1 handful of spinach (Juice together)

• 2 slices of raw sprouted bread (Don't toast, NO butter)
• 1 salad…
  - 3 lg kale leaves cut into bite size pieces (stems
    removed)
  - 1 1/2 cups red cabbage diced
  - 1 cup julienne carrots
  - 1/2 cup pecans

Dressing:

• 1 Tbs apple cider vinegar
• 2 Tbs first cold pressed olive oil
• 1 tsp thyme
• sea salt to taste (optional)

Mix kale, cabbage, carrots, and pecans in a medium salad bowl. Add apple cider vinegar, olive oil, thyme, and salt (if using) and toss well. Enjoy!

SNACK

• 1 glass of water
• 1 pear or fruit of your choice
• 1 cup peppermint or herbal tea (add honey for flavor)

DINNER

• 1 glass of water
• 1 slice of raw sprouted bread (Don't toast, NO butter)
• 1 Raw Thai Soup…
  - 2 celery stalks roughly chopped
  - 1 garlic clove
  - 2 kaffir lime leaves
  - 2 Tbs coconut oil

- 3 Tbs cold pressed olive oil
- sea salt to taste (optional)
- 2 cups of water

Blend all together until smooth. Pour into a medium bowl and add…

1 head baby bok choy sliced
3/4 cup roughly chopped broccoli florets
1/2 cup quartered cherry tomatoes
1/2 cup avocado diced
1/4 cup cilantro leaves

Enjoy!

DAY 14

BREAKFAST

- 1 glass of water
- 1 glass of juice…
    - About 1/2 cup of roughly chopped pineapple
    - About a 2 inch piece of cucumber
    - 1 handful of spinach
    - 1 reg size apple
    - 3 reg size carrots

Juice them up and enjoy!

- 1 bowl of homemade oatmeal…

Bring 2 cups of water to a boil. Then add 3/4 cup of oatmeal, 1 dash of sea salt, a dash of cinnamon powder or about an inch of a cinnamon stick, and 2-3 Tbs of honey. Oats are ready once it starts to boil. *Enjoy!*

SNACK

- 1 glass of water
- 1 banana with about 1/2 tsp peanut butter for each bite
- 1 12oz glass of organic soy milk

LUNCH

- 1 glass of water
- 1 glass of fresh juice…
    - 1 lg orange
    - About a 2 inch piece of sweet potato

- About 1/2 cup roughly chopped jicama
- 1 lg celery stalk
- 1 lg green apple

Juice them up and squeeze 1/2 lime into it (about 1 tbs). *Enjoy!*

• 1 slice of raw sprouted bread (Don't toast, NO butter)
• 1 salad…
- 2 lg kale leaves cut into bite size pieces
- 3 lg romaine lettuce leaves cut into bite size pieces
- 1 cup sliced red cabbage
- 2 tbs dried cherries
- ¼ cup walnuts
- ¼ cup Bragg Ginger and Sesame dressing
- 2 tsp hemp seeds

Mix kale, lettuce, cabbage, cherries, and walnuts together. Toss with Bragg Ginger and Sesame dressing, and sprinkle with hemp seeds. Enjoy!

SNACK

1 glass of water
1 12oz glass of Kombucha
1 bowl of fruit, nuts, and Raw Organic Kefir for probiotics;
- ½ apple diced
- ½ orange diced
- ½ sliced banana
- 2 tbs chopped almonds
- 2 tbs chopped cashews
- 2 tbs pecans
- 2 tbs Raw Organic Kefir

In a bowl combine apple, orange, and banana. Top with kefir and sprinkle chopped nuts and pecans on top. Enjoy!

DINNER

- 1 glass of water
- 1 cup ACV tea
- 1 slice of raw sprouted bread (Don't toast, NO butter)
- 1 Raw Sweet Corn Soup…
    - ¾ cup sweet corn kernels
    - ¼ cup walnuts
    - 2 Tbs first cold pressed olive oil
    - ½ tsp fresh garlic
    - sea salt to taste (optional)
    - 1 cup water

Blend all together until smooth. Pour into a medium bowl and add…

1/2 cup sweet corn kernels
1/4 cup diced avocado
1/4 cup diced red bell pepper
2 tbs cilantro leaves
1/2 tsp fresh cracked black pepper

Enjoy!

DAY 15

BREAKFAST

- 1 glass of water
- 1 bowl of cereal…
    - 1 cup of organic raw oatmeal
    - 1/2 cup of your favorite healthy cereal
    - 1 sliced banana
    - 1 1/2 cup of almond milk
    - Honey to taste (optional)

In a cereal bowl mix oatmeal and cereal. Slice a banana and pour the milk into it. (Top with a swirl of honey)

SNACK

- 1 glass of water
- 1 kiwi
- 1 orange

Eat kiwi and orange raw

LUNCH

- 1 glass of water
- 1 cup ACV tea (recipe on page 100)
- 1 glass of juice…
    - 1 medium roma tomato
    - 2 medium carrots
    - About 1/4 cup broccoli
    - 1 piece of garlic

- About 3 inch piece of cucumber
- 1/2 lime (about 1 tbs of juice once squeezed)

Juice the tomato, carrots, broccoli, garlic, and cucumber. Squeeze the fresh lime juice and enjoy!

• 1 Raw Herb Pizza with baked crust…

4oz whole grain mix pizza crust (my wife and I like the wheat, gluten, and dairy free pizza crust powder from our health food store). Prepare and spread as directed on the label of the bag but bake at 350°F. for about 15-20 minutes or until light brown. Then top with Macadamia Cheese, Sun-dried Tomato Sauce, and Toppings…

Macadamia Cheese
• 1/4 cup macadamia nuts
• 1/2 tbs lemon juice
• 1 clove garlic
• 1/4 cup basil leaves
• sea salt to taste (optional)
• water as needed

Blend all together adding only enough water to make a smooth creamy texture.

Cont…
Sun-dried Tomato Sauce…

• 1/2 cup roughly chopped tomatoes
• 1/2 tsp fresh garlic
• 1/4 cup basil leaves
• 1 tsp first cold pressed olive oil
• 1/2 tsp fresh lemon juice
• 2 pitted dates

- 1/2 tsp fresh oregano
- 1/4 tsp fresh rosemary
- sea salt to taste (optional)1tbs sun-dried tomatoes

Blend tomatoes, garlic, basil, oil, lemon juice, dates, oregano, rosemary, and salt (if using) until smooth. Add the sun-dried tomatoes and blend until mixed well.

Toppings
- 1/2 sm tomato thinly sliced
- 1 1/2 tbs pitted and sliced black olives
- 2 tbs sun-dried tomatoes sliced
- 1 tsp fresh oregano leaves
- 1/4 cup fresh basil leaves

Enjoy!

SNACK

- 1 glass of water
- 1/2 cup of diced watermelon
- 1/2 cup of cantaloupe

DINNER

- 1 glass of water
- 1 cup ACV tea (recipe on page 100)
- 1 slice of raw sprouted bread (Don't toast, NO butter)
- 1 Salad…
    - 3 cups mix of baby greens
    - 1/2 cup julienne orange bell pepper
    - 1/2 cup julienne beets
    - 1/4 cup quartered cherry tomatoes

- 1 Tbs of hemp seeds
- 2-3 Tbs of Bragg Ginger and Sesame dressing

Mix the greens, bell pepper, beets, and tomatoes. Toss with dressing and sprinkle with hemp seeds. Enjoy!

DAY 16

BREAKFAST

• 1 glass of water
• 1 bowl of fruit, nuts, and Raw Organic Kefir for probiotics;
        - 1 apple cored and diced
        - 2 Tbs dried cranberries
        - 2 Tbs raw pepitas
        - 1/4 cup diced mango
        - 1/4 cup kefir
        - 1 tbs flax seeds
        - 1 tbs black sesame seeds

In a bowl combine apple, cranberries, pepitas, and mango. Top with kefir and sprinkle with flax and sesame seeds. Enjoy!

SNACK

• 1 glass of water
• 1 cup of grapes
• 1/4 cup of almonds

Eat snacks raw

LUNCH

• 1 glass of water
• 1 slice of raw sprouted bread (Don't toast, NO butter)
• 1 Glass of Fresh Juice

- 1 apple
- 1 orange
- 3 carrots
- 1 cup fresh spinach leaves
- 2 leaves of kale (stems removed)
- 1 small beet
- 1 slice of ginger (size of a US quarter)

Juice them up and enjoy!

• 1 Bowl of Veggie Lentil Soup

Recipe makes about 4 bowls

• 8 cups water
• 1 cup lentils
• 1 Tbs olive oil
• ½ cup chopped onion
• 1 tsp minced fresh garlic
• 1 Lg roma tomato
• 3 reg size roughly chopped carrots
• 2 reg size roughly chopped celery stalks
• 1 reg bunch of green chard cut into bite size
• sea salt and pepper to taste

In a large pot bring the water to boil. Add the lentils, bring to boil, put the lid on and lower to medium-low heat and simmer until lentils are al dente (15 minutes or so) While the lentils cook, heat the oil in a medium skillet over medium-low heat. Add the onion and garlic and sauté for 3-5 minutes then add the tomato and sauté until the it has become like a sauce.

Check the lentils. If they are al dente, add the "sauce",

carrots, celery, chard, salt and pepper to the pot and simmer with lid on for 10-15 minutes more. Enjoy!

SNACK

- 1 glass of water
- 1 cup diced pineapple
- 1 peach

DINNER

- 1 glass of water
- 1 cup ACV tea (recipe on page 100)
- 1 Colorful Salad…
    - About 5 Romaine lettuce leaves cut into bite size
    - 1/4 cup julienne carrots
    - 1/4 cup fresh tomato diced
    - 1/4 cup fresh cucumber diced
    - 1/4 cup broccoli florets
    - 1 Tbs apple cider vinegar
    - 2 Tbs olive oil
    - Sea salt to taste (optional)

In a large bowl mix romaine lettuce, carrots, tomato, cucumber, and broccoli. Add vinegar, olive oil and salt (if using), and mix again. Enjoy!

About The Author

Nathan Crane is a natural health researcher and certified holistic cancer coach. He is an award-winning author, inspirational speaker, Amazon #1 bestselling author and 20x award-winning documentary filmmaker.Nathan is on the Board of Directors for the Beljanski Foundation, a Non-Profit Conducting Scientific Research into Natural Solutions for Cancer.

Nathan is also the Director of Healing Life, President of the Holistic Leadership Council, Founder of Conquering Cancer, and Director and Producer of the award winning documentary film, Cancer; The Integrative Perspective. Nathan has received numerous awards including the Accolade 2020 Outstanding Achievement Humanitarian Award, and the Outstanding Community Service Award from the California Senate for his work in education and empowerment with natural and integrative methods for healing cancer.

You can receive a Free Download of his bestselling book absolutely free by visiting BecomingCancerFree.com
To share your experience about The Panacea Cleanse,

upload a video of you talking about the cleanse to

Youtube and title it "The Panacea Cleanse then email the

link to info@thepanaceacommunity.com